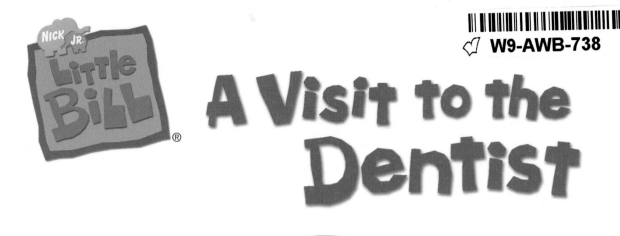

A Visit to the Dentist

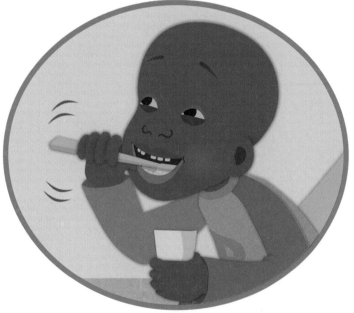

by Eleanor Fremont

illustrated by Andy Mastrocinque

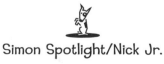

Simon Spotlight/Nick Jr.

New York   London   Toronto   Sydney   Singapore

Based on the TV series *Little Bill*® created by Bill Cosby as seen on Nick Jr.®

SIMON SPOTLIGHT
An imprint of Simon & Schuster Children's Publishing Division
1230 Avenue of the Americas, New York, New York 10020
Manufactured in the United States of America
First Edition   10 9 8 7 6 5 4 3 2 1
ISBN 0-689-84632-0

"Remember, Little Bill," said his mother, Brenda, one day at breakfast, "I'm taking you to the dentist after school today."

"The dentist?" Little Bill asked. He had forgotten all about his dentist appointment. "My tummy feels funny."

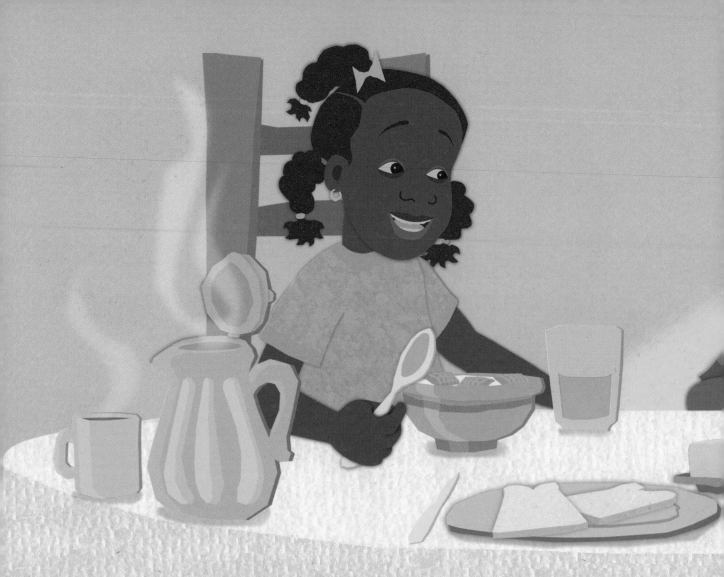

"Are you worried about seeing the dentist?" asked Bobby.

"I don't think so," said Little Bill. But his tummy still felt funny.

"Remember what they do there?" asked April. "You get to go up and down in the big chair."

"And they take an X ray and clean your teeth with a buzzy toothbrush," said Bobby.

"Oh, yeah!" said Little Bill. "The one that goes bzzz, bzzz!"

By the time April and Bobby had finished talking, Little Bill's tummy felt much better.

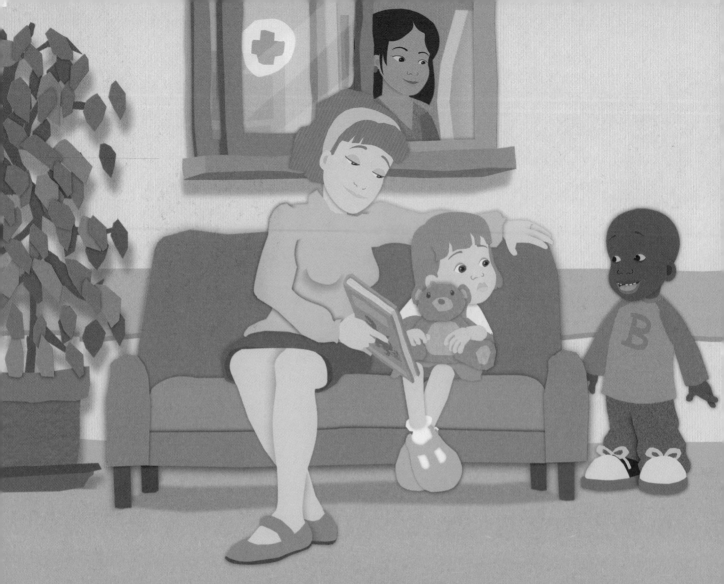

That afternoon when Little Bill and Brenda got to the dentist's office, there was a little girl in the waiting room. She held her teddy bear tight.

"Want to read a book, Marlene?" asked the little girl's mother.

"Nope," said Marlene. She squeezed her bear even tighter.

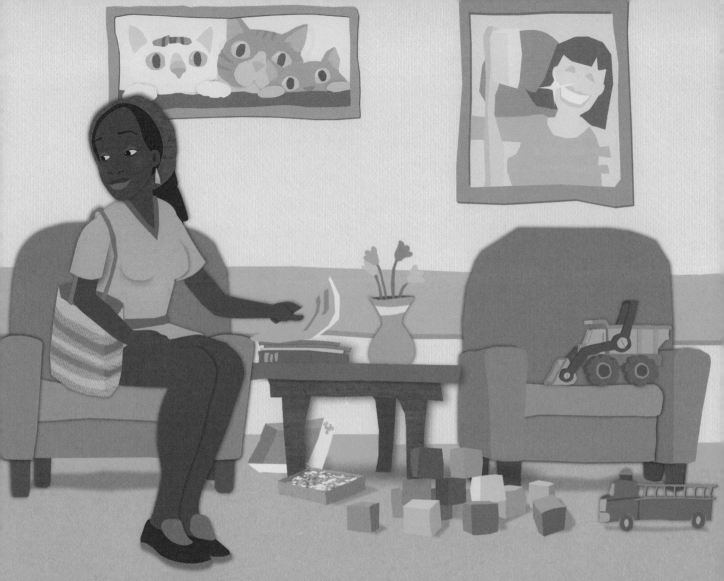

Little Bill went over to her. "Are you scared about seeing the dentist?" he asked.

"My bear's a little scared," said Marlene. "But I'm not."

Little Bill thought she looked scared, though.

"It's Marlene's first visit," her mother explained.

Kelly, the dental assistant, came out to get Little Bill. "Ready?" she asked.

"Ready," said Little Bill.

In they went. Little Bill sat down in the big chair. "Can you make it go up and down?" he asked Kelly.

"Sure!" Kelly said with a laugh.

Next Kelly looked at Little Bill's teeth with a small mirror and counted every one of them.

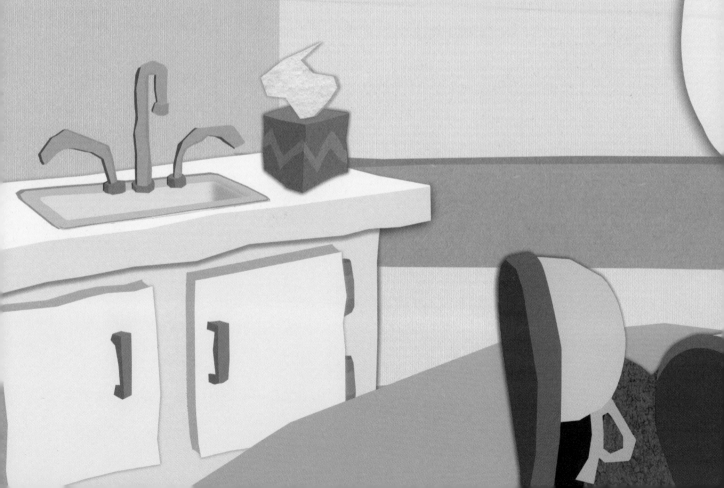

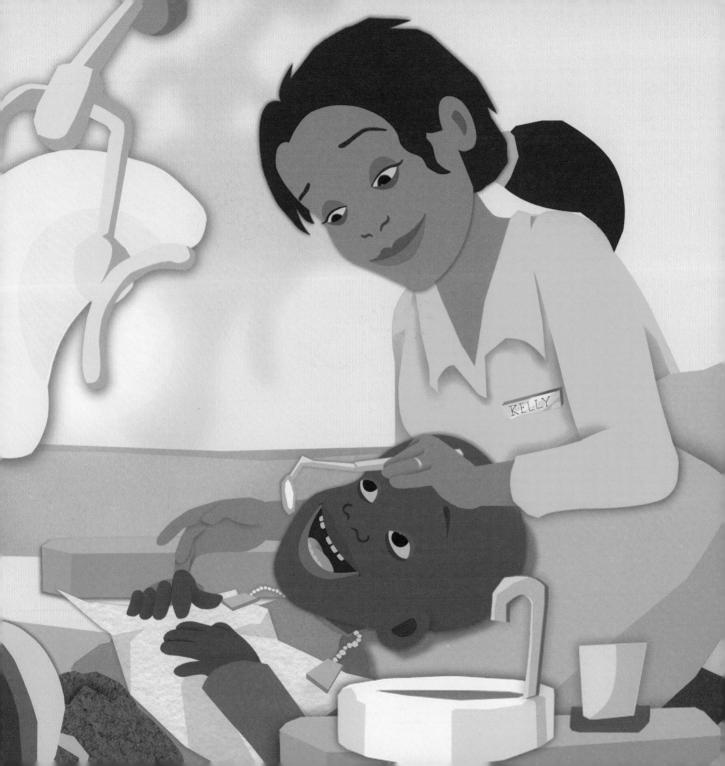

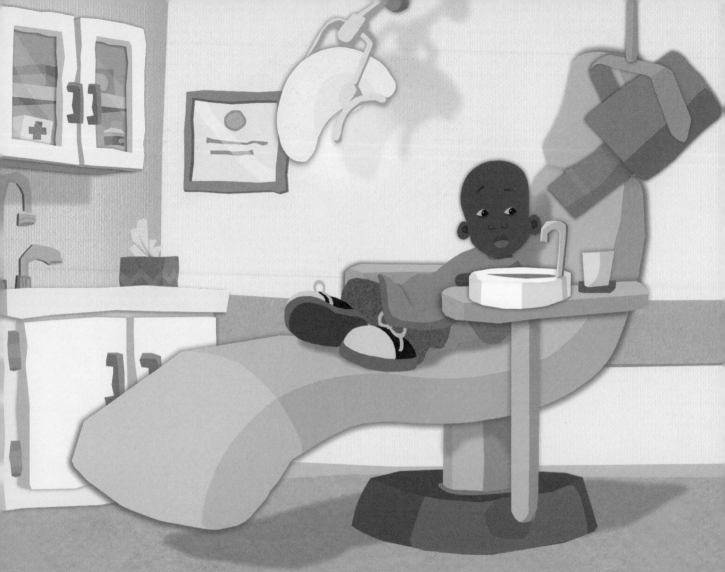

"Now I'm going to give your teeth an X ray," she said. "Do you remember what that is, Little Bill?"

"Uh-huh. It's a picture of my teeth," he said.

"That's right. It's a picture of your teeth growing inside your gums."

"Is it going to hurt?" Little Bill asked, starting to feel a little worried.

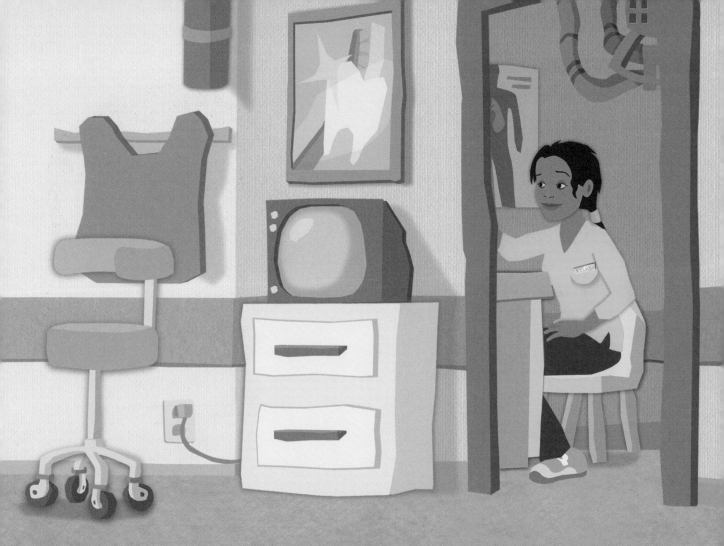

"Don't worry, Little Bill. Nothing will hurt. I'm going out of the room to work the machine, okay?"

Kelly left the room for a second. Little Bill heard a clicking noise, and then Kelly came back in. Nothing hurt at all.

Then Dr. Jackson came in and looked at Little Bill's X rays.

"Those are all my teeth!" Little Bill exclaimed when Dr. Jackson showed him the pictures.

"Yes," Dr. Jackson said, "and they are very healthy teeth."

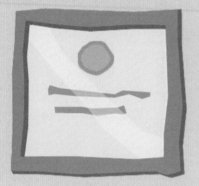

Then she cleaned Little Bill's teeth with a tickly electric toothbrush. "Time to rinse," Dr. Jackson said, holding out a little paper cup. "Now, Little Bill," said Dr. Jackson, "can you show me how you brush your teeth in circles?" Little Bill showed her and she smiled. "Great job! You're a very good patient, Little Bill!"

"Don't forget to take a sticker before you leave," Kelly said.

"I won't!" said Little Bill as he picked out a special dinosaur sticker for himself. "The dinosaur's teeth look very healthy!" Little Bill said, giggling.

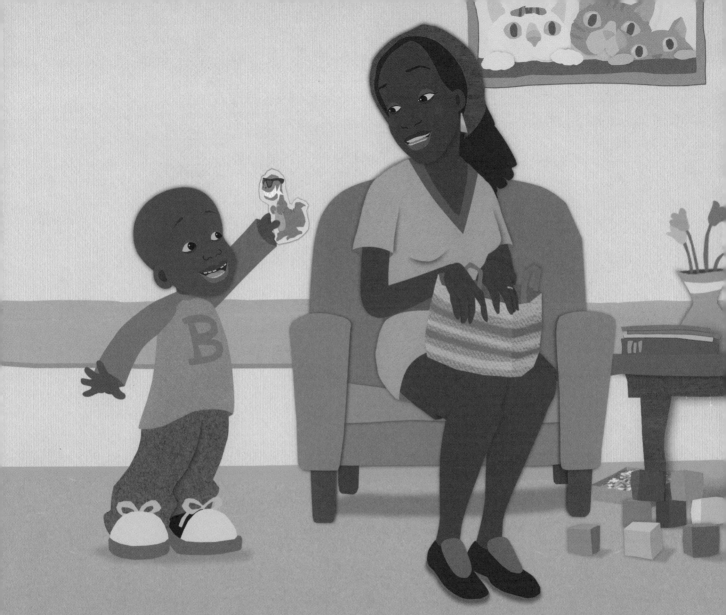

"How was it?" Brenda asked him when he came out.

"It was just the way Bobby and April told me it would be. And I got a sticker!"

"That's a very nice sticker, Little Bill," said Brenda.

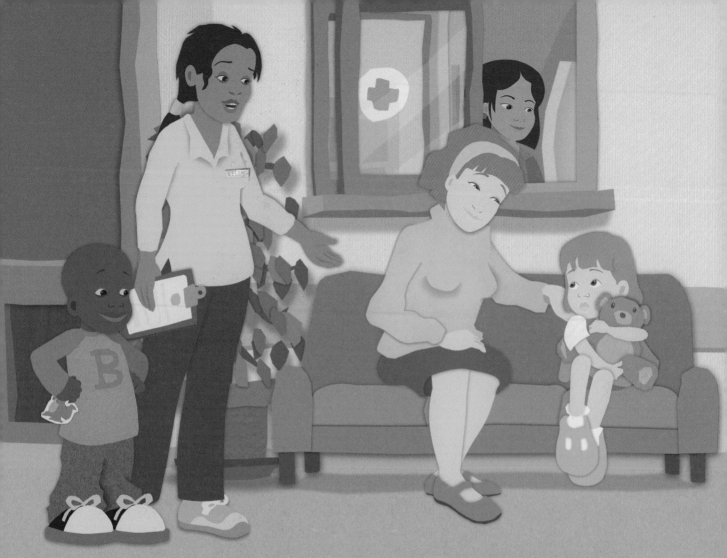

"Your turn, Marlene," said Kelly. But Marlene didn't budge.

Little Bill tugged on Kelly's sleeve. "I think her bear's afraid," he whispered.

Kelly smiled. "I'll tell you what, Little Bill. Maybe you could show Marlene's bear what it's like?"

"Okay," said Little Bill. He felt very important.

Little Bill sat Marlene's bear down in the dentist's chair. "What's his name?" he asked Marlene.

"Oscar," she replied.

"Oscar, do you want to take a ride up and down in the chair?" Little Bill asked.

Marlene made Oscar's head nod.

"Here we go," said Little Bill. Kelly made the chair go up and down.

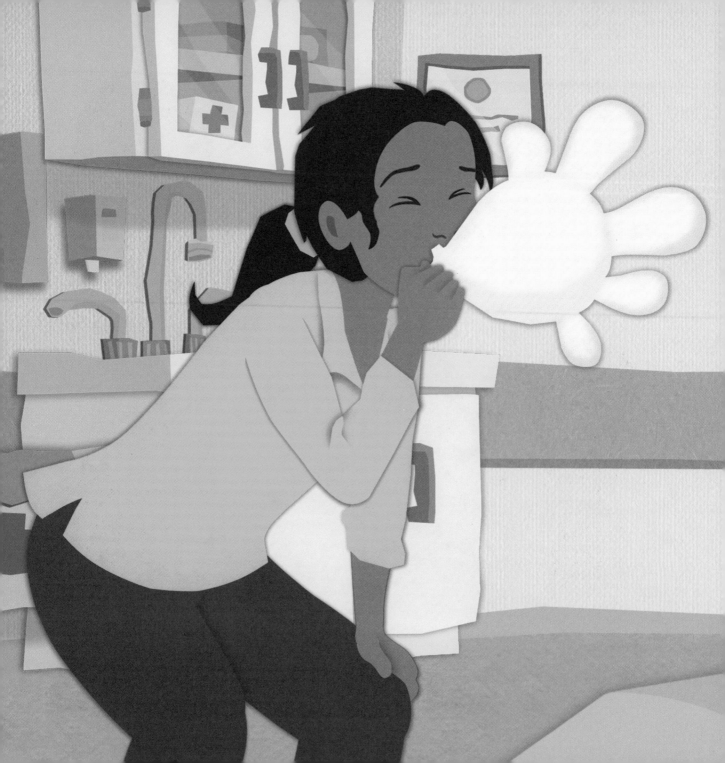

"Oscar liked that," said Marlene.

"Wait until you see this, Oscar," said Kelly. She took out a thin, white rubber glove and blew it up like a balloon.

"Wow!" exclaimed Marlene.

"Now you can count Oscar's teeth," Kelly told Little Bill.

So he pretended to count Oscar's teeth. "Five zillion!" he said. "That's a lot of teeth!"

Marlene laughed.

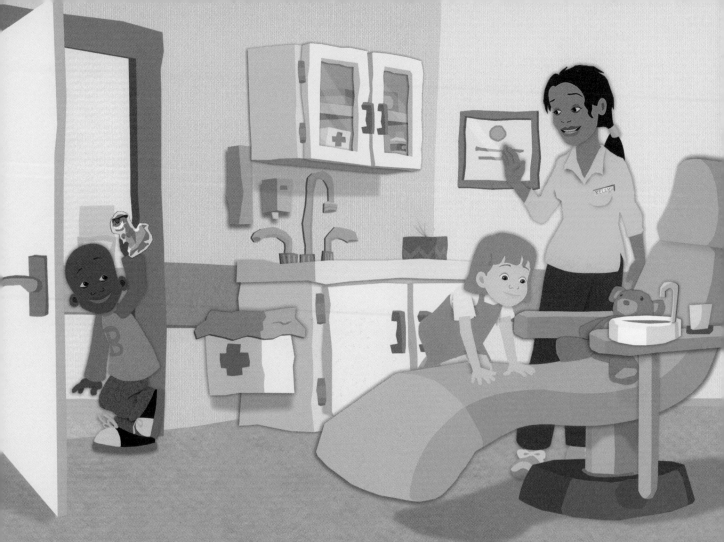

"All right, Oscar, you're all done," said Kelly. "He was a very good patient, and you're a great bear dentist, Little Bill."

Little Bill was very proud of himself.

"Ready for your checkup?" Kelly asked Marlene.

"Yes!" said Marlene. "Can I get a sticker at the end too?"

Kelly laughed. "Of course you can!"

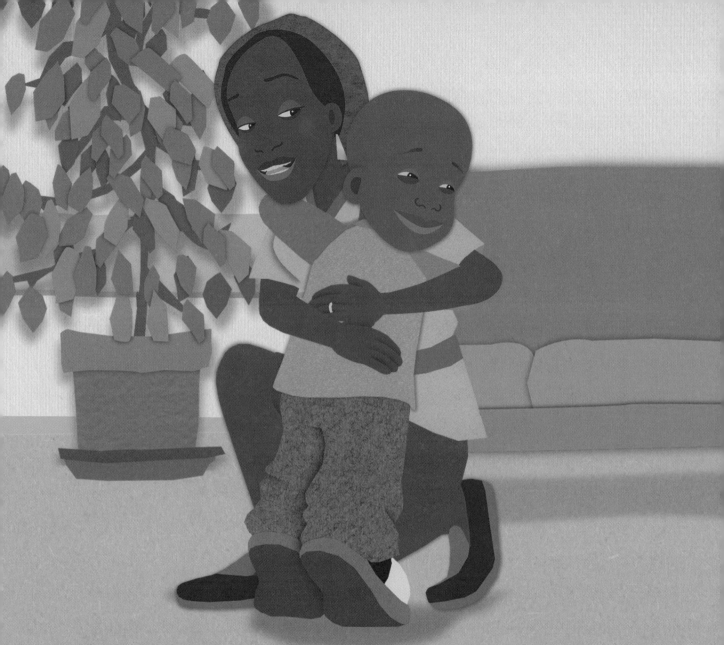

When Brenda saw Little Bill come out she gave him a hug. "That was very nice of you," she said.

"Now Marlene won't be scared of the dentist anymore," said Little Bill.

"How was the dentist today?" Little Bill's dad asked at dinner that night.

"It was fun," said Little Bill. "I helped a girl named Marlene because she was scared. Dr. Jackson said my teeth are very healthy, and I got a dinosaur sticker, too!"

"And guess what I want to be when I grow up," Little Bill added.

"Let me guess . . .," Bobby said.

"A dentist?"

"Nope!" Little Bill exclaimed. "A bear dentist!"
And everyone laughed and laughed.